# Where Did All the Teachers Go?

By Nancy Villabona
Interviews With Children on COVID-19

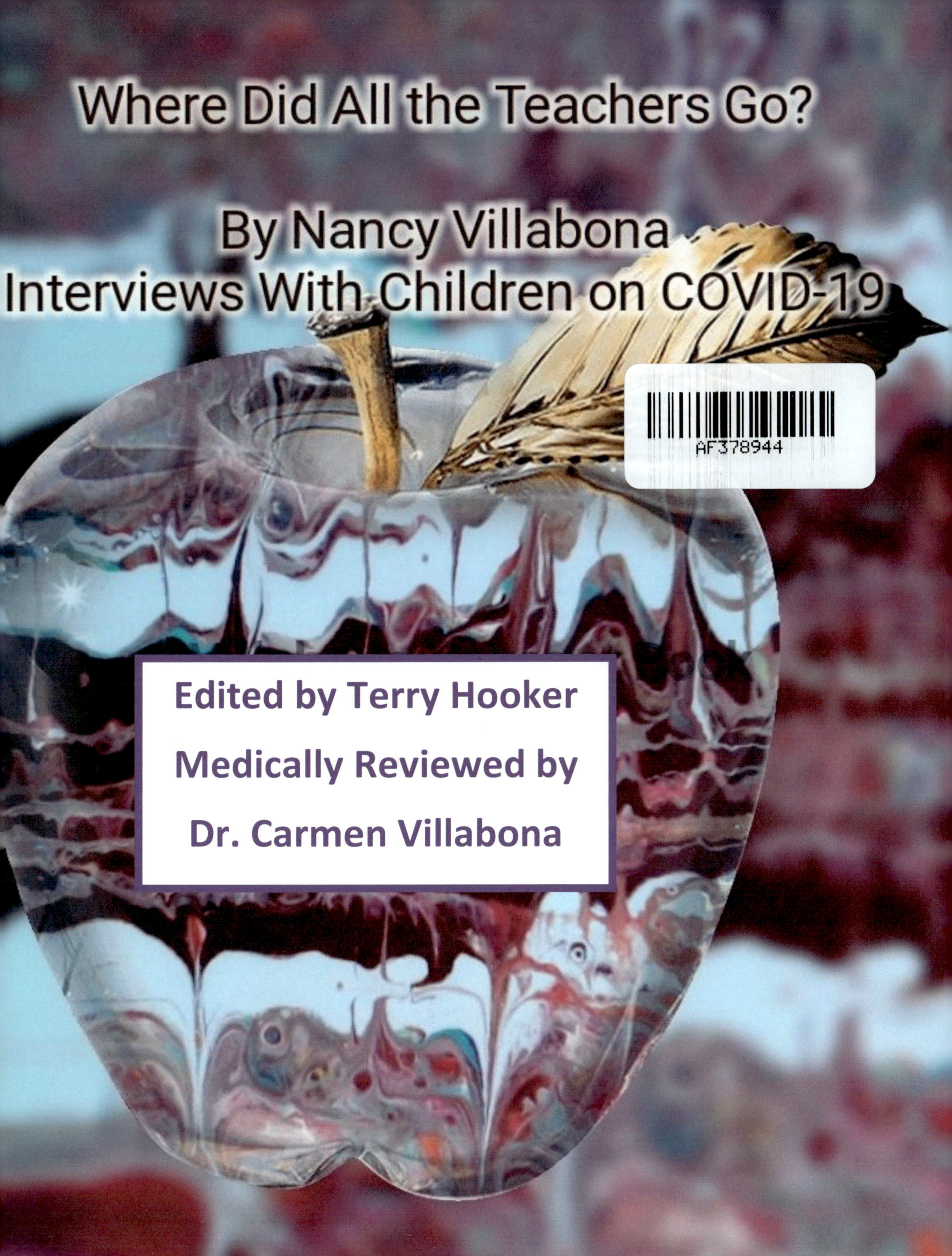

Edited by Terry Hooker

Medically Reviewed by

Dr. Carmen Villabona

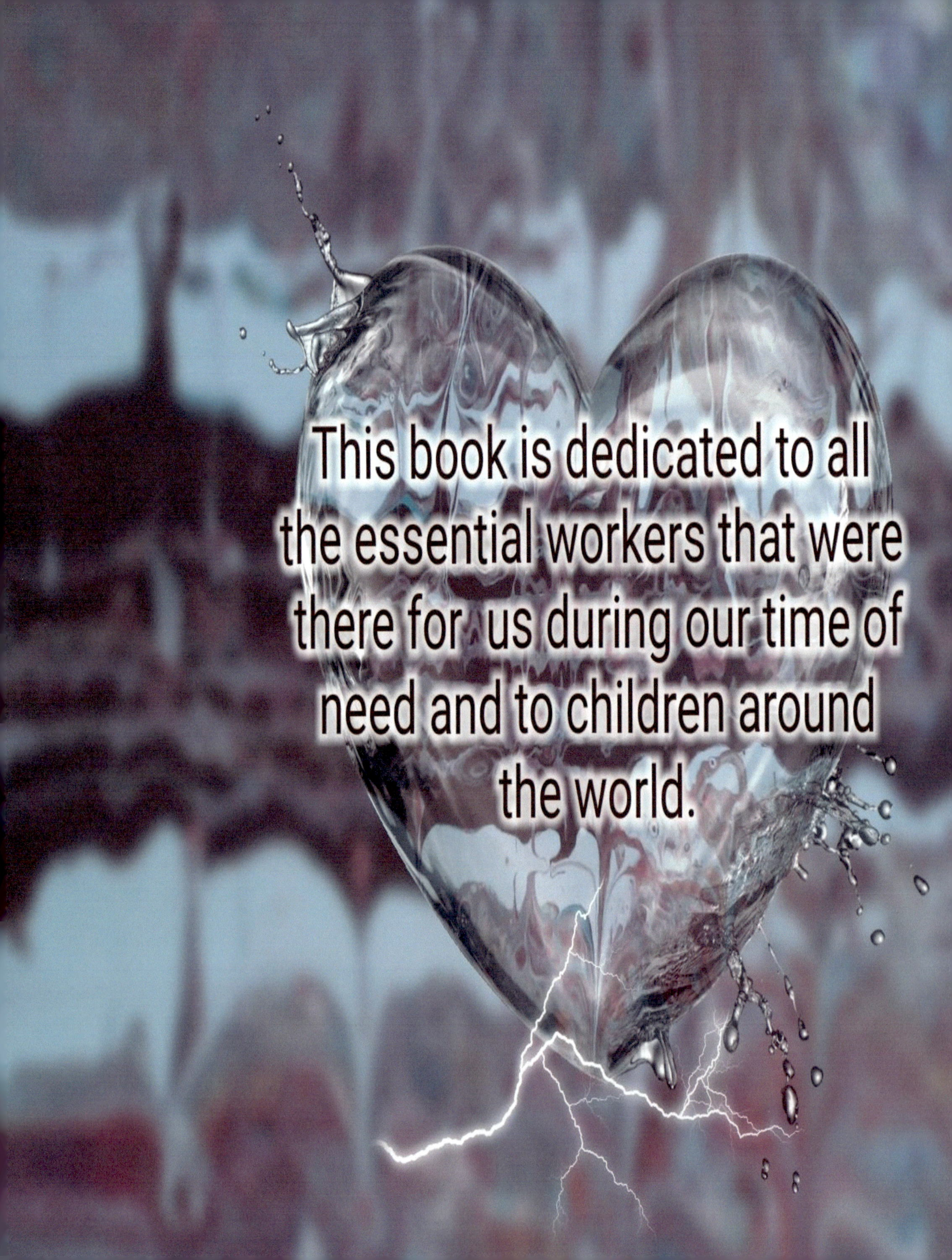

This book is dedicated to all the essential workers that were there for  us during our time of need and to children around the world.

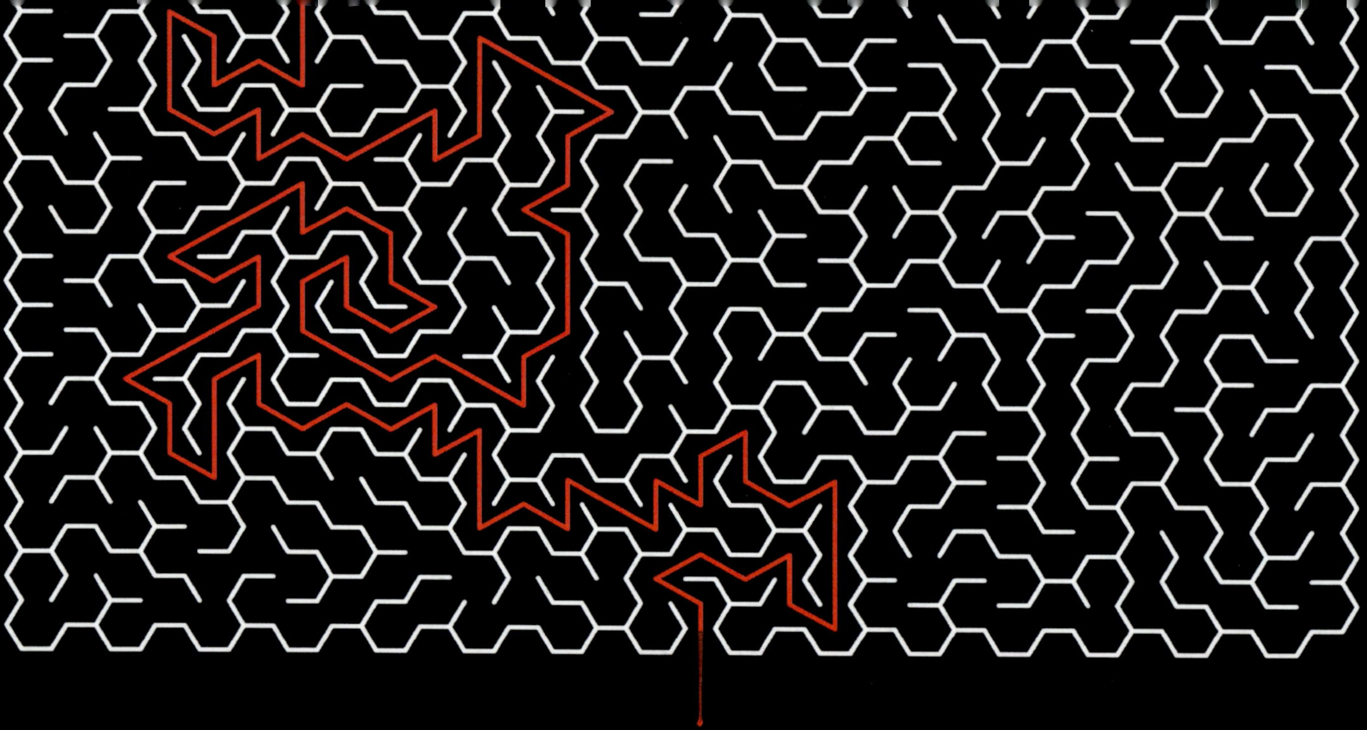

# HARTE
# SPIELE

Labyrinthe Für Erwachsene

ActivityCrusades
activity books

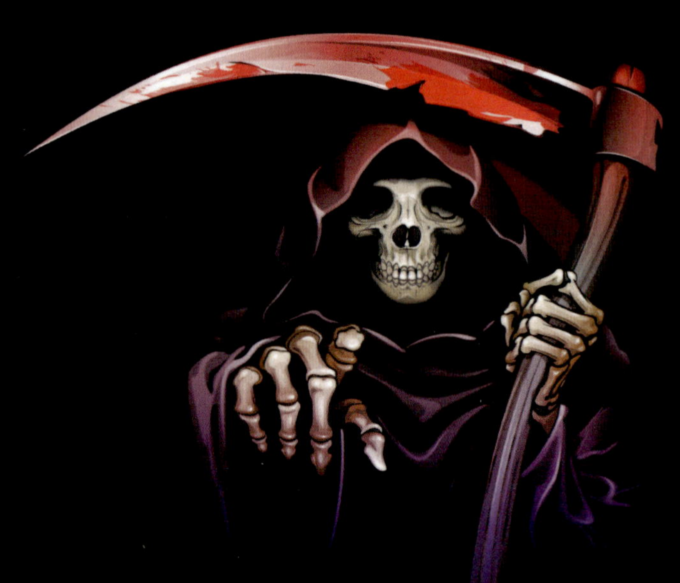

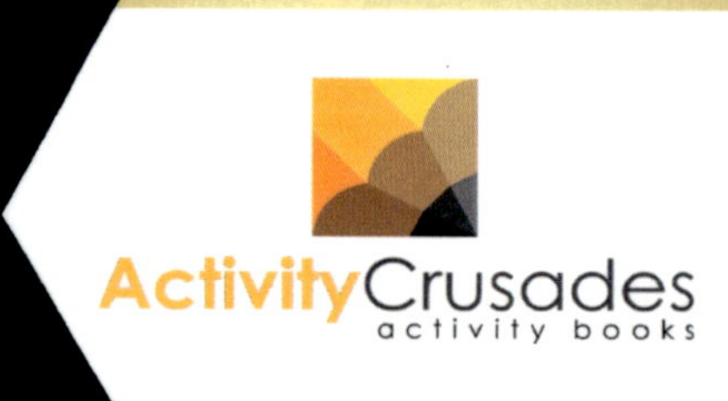

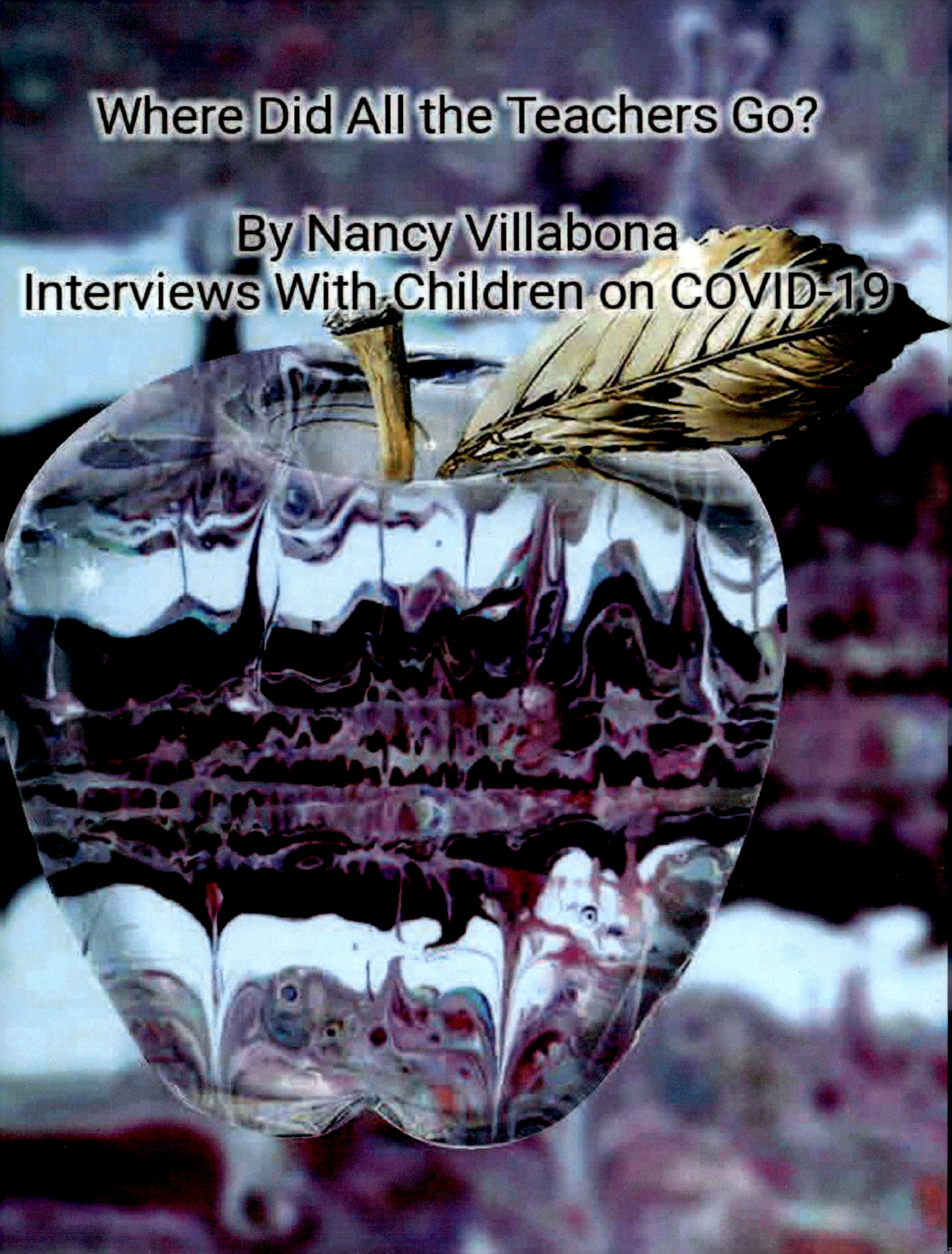

Where Did All the Teachers Go?

By Nancy Villabona
Interviews With Children on COVID-19

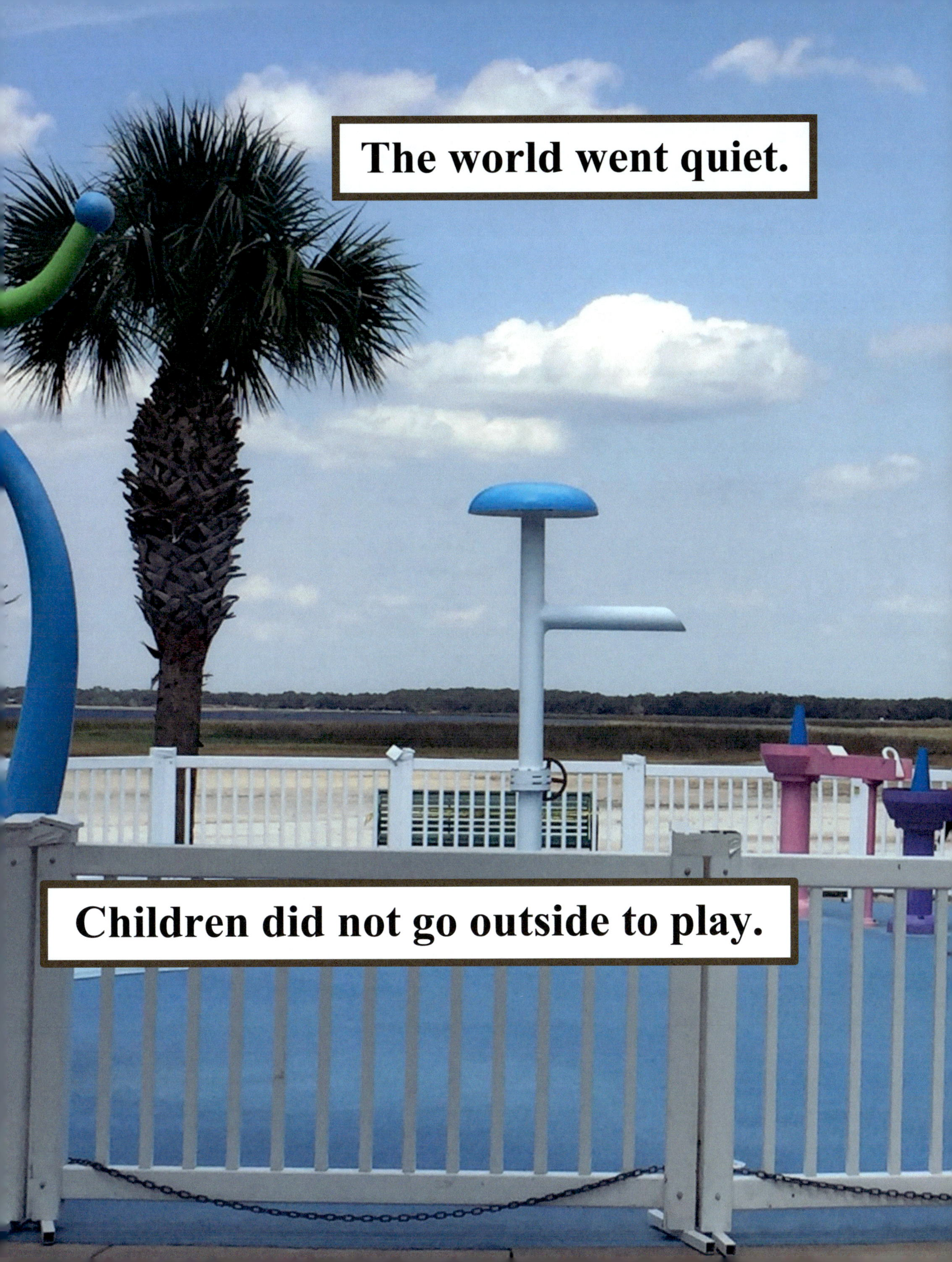
The world went quiet.
Children did not go outside to play.

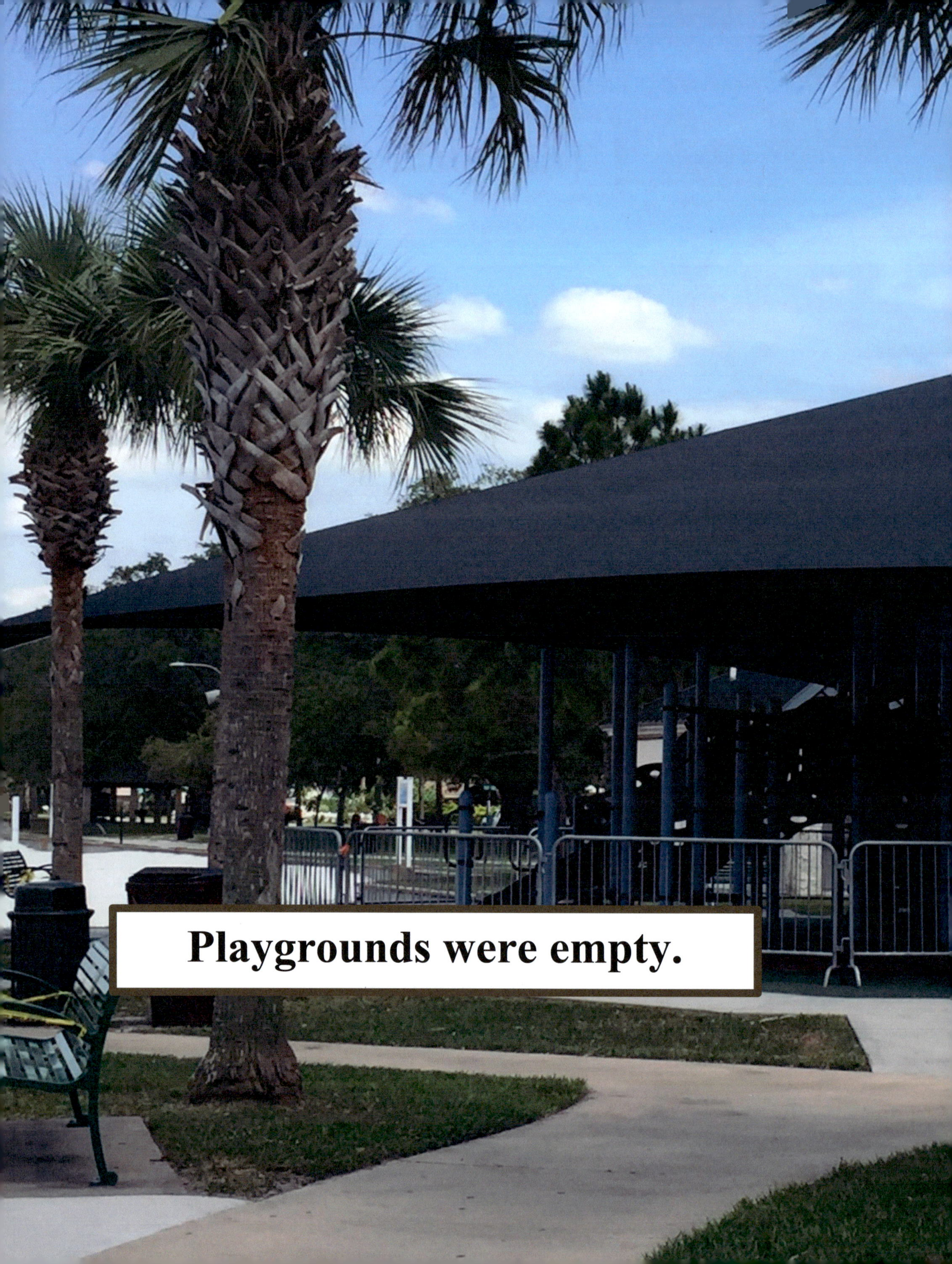
Playgrounds were empty.

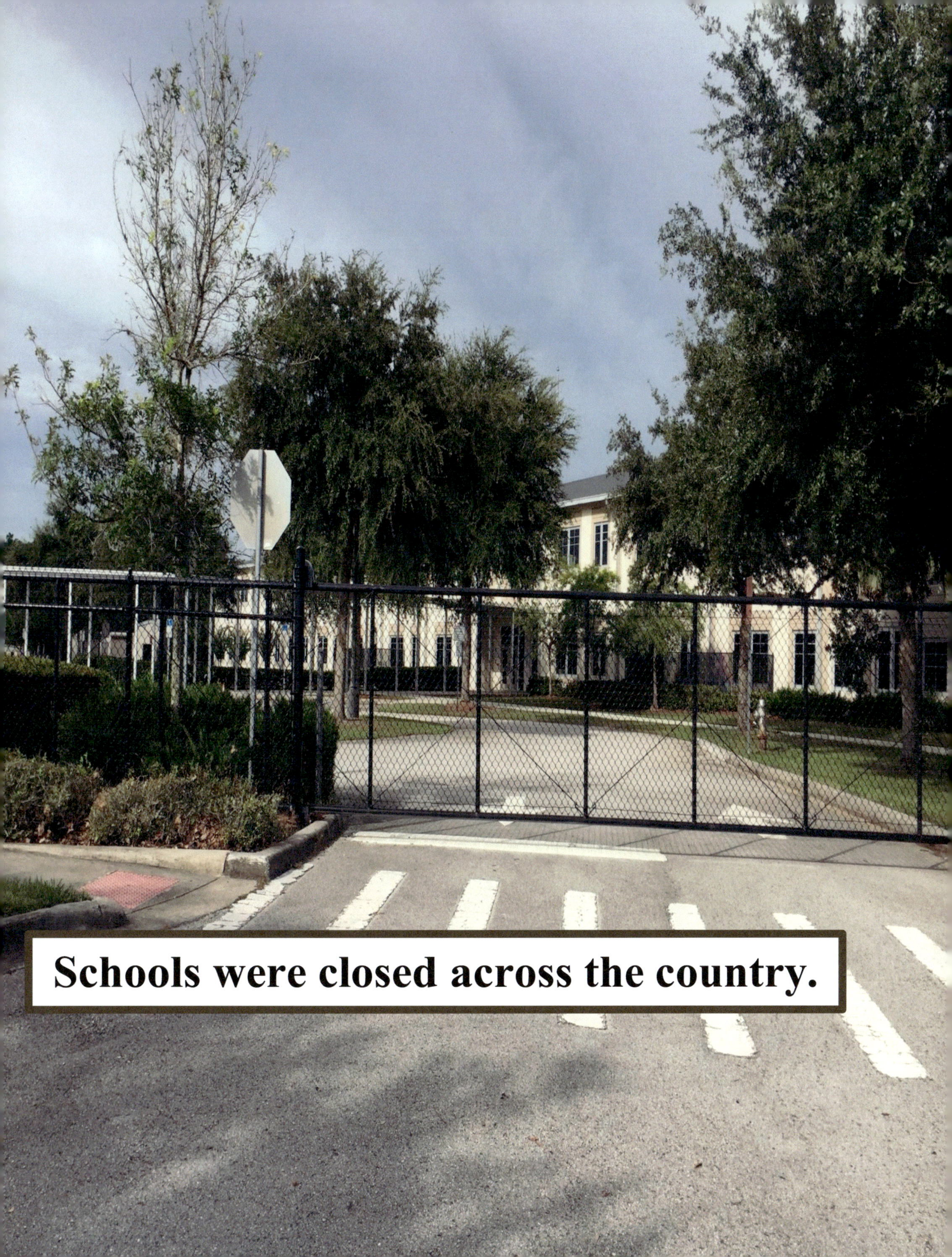

Schools were closed across the country.

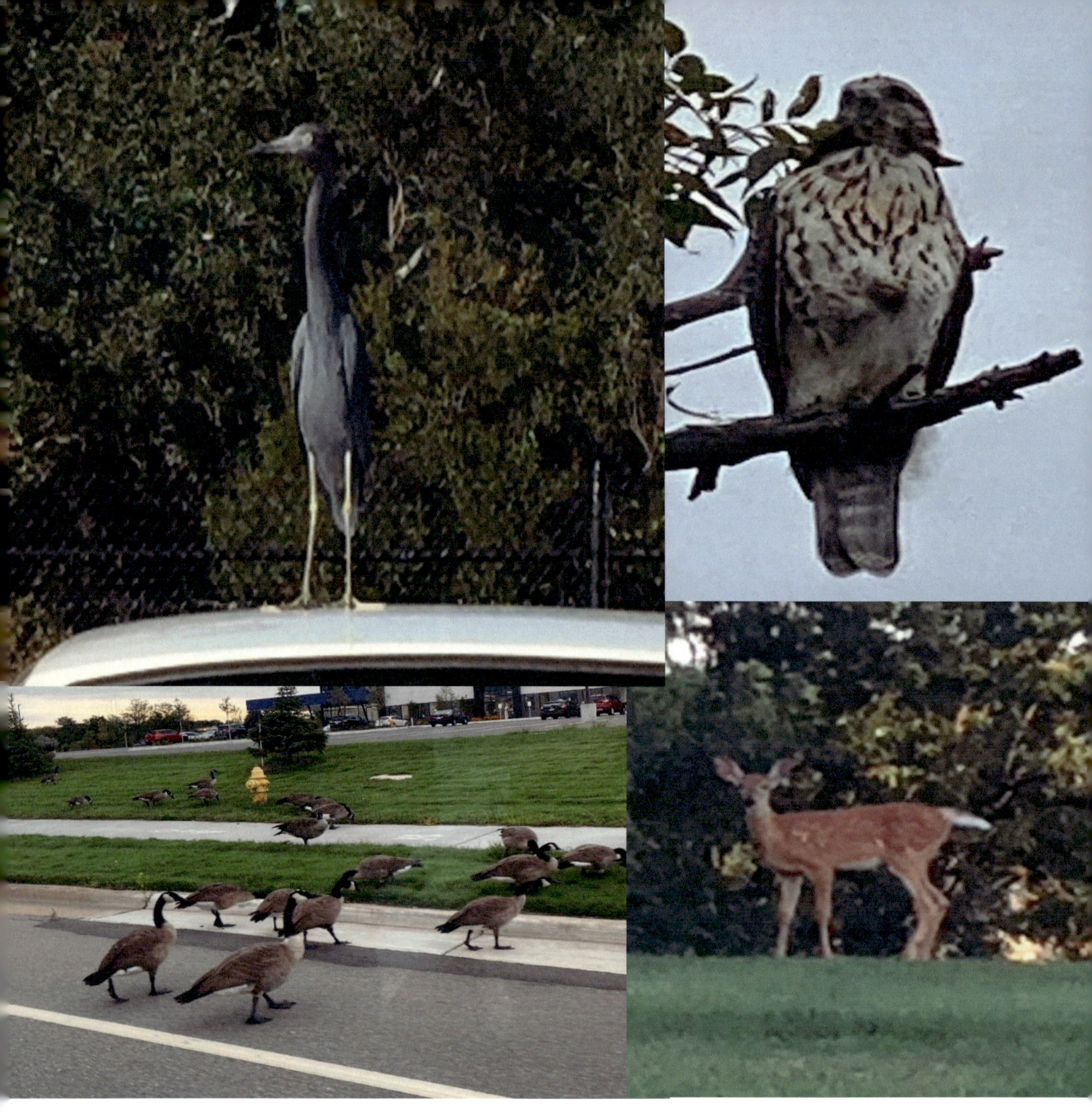

Deer, birds, and other creatures began to wander into yards as if searching for lost friends.

*COVID-19, otherwise known as The Corona Virus, or The Pandemic,* appeared in 2020.

## Our world was rocked.

## Life as we knew it changed.

## How did the children feel?

## What were the children thinking?

With parental consent, interviews with children were conducted. Ages of the children were posted as the age when they were first interviewed. The children were asked the same five questions.

Please note that these questions were asked just as the *COVID-19* Virus was coming out.

Information on *What We Know* information was constantly changing, so, *What We Know* responses to the questions were current at the time of the response but may have changed since printing. Check with the *Center for Disease Control (CDC):* for the most current information in the United States of America.

# Question 1: What do you want to know about the virus?

**Viviana 5, West Palm Beach, FL: I want to know about the sickness.**

**Elena 7, Stockholm, Sweden, Sydney 6, Dayton, MN: How dangerous is it and what can happen?**

What we know: It is called *COVID-19. The Corona Virus* and it is a *pandemic.* It is an airborne virus.

What we know: It can be dangerous for the elderly people that have underlying conditions such as cancer, obesity, diabetes, or other conditions that cause their body to be weakened. People can get ill. Some may die. Children are less likely to get sick unless they have a weakened immune system or underlying condition. Children may show signs of rashes, low blood pressure, diarrhea, tiredness, flu like symptoms and rare cases children have gotten an inflammatory syndrome called

MIS-C. (Multisystem Inflammatory Syndrome in Children) *

**Carmen 9, Weston, FL:  Could I get the virus?**

**Luke 11: Spokane, WA: Does it make you sick?**

What we know: Yes, children can get the virus. Children that may have other illnesses are more likely to display symptoms. You could have no *symptoms* (they call that *asymptomatic*) or a few. Fever, *fatigue*, coughs, breathing difficulties, tightening of chest, low oxygen levels are some symptoms you may experience.

## Can the virus be transmitted to animals?

What we know: Yes, Pets get *COVID-19* by close contact with people affected with *COVID-19*.



What we know: Take precautions not to expose yourself or animals to the virus. Wash your hands before and after being with your pet. Pets can test positive. They may show no symptoms, or they may become sick. Symptoms may include: Coughing, sneezing, or weakness.

* There is a vaccination for pets.



What we know: We do not have a timeline for when it will end. Vaccines hopefully will slow the spread, but variants (changes to the virus) are still appearing. This may mean that we will never get rid of COVID-19, we may need to vaccinate yearly, just like some get a flu shot every year, although this has not been determined at the publishing of this book.

***See the *CDC Guidelines* for more specific information on people and pets.**

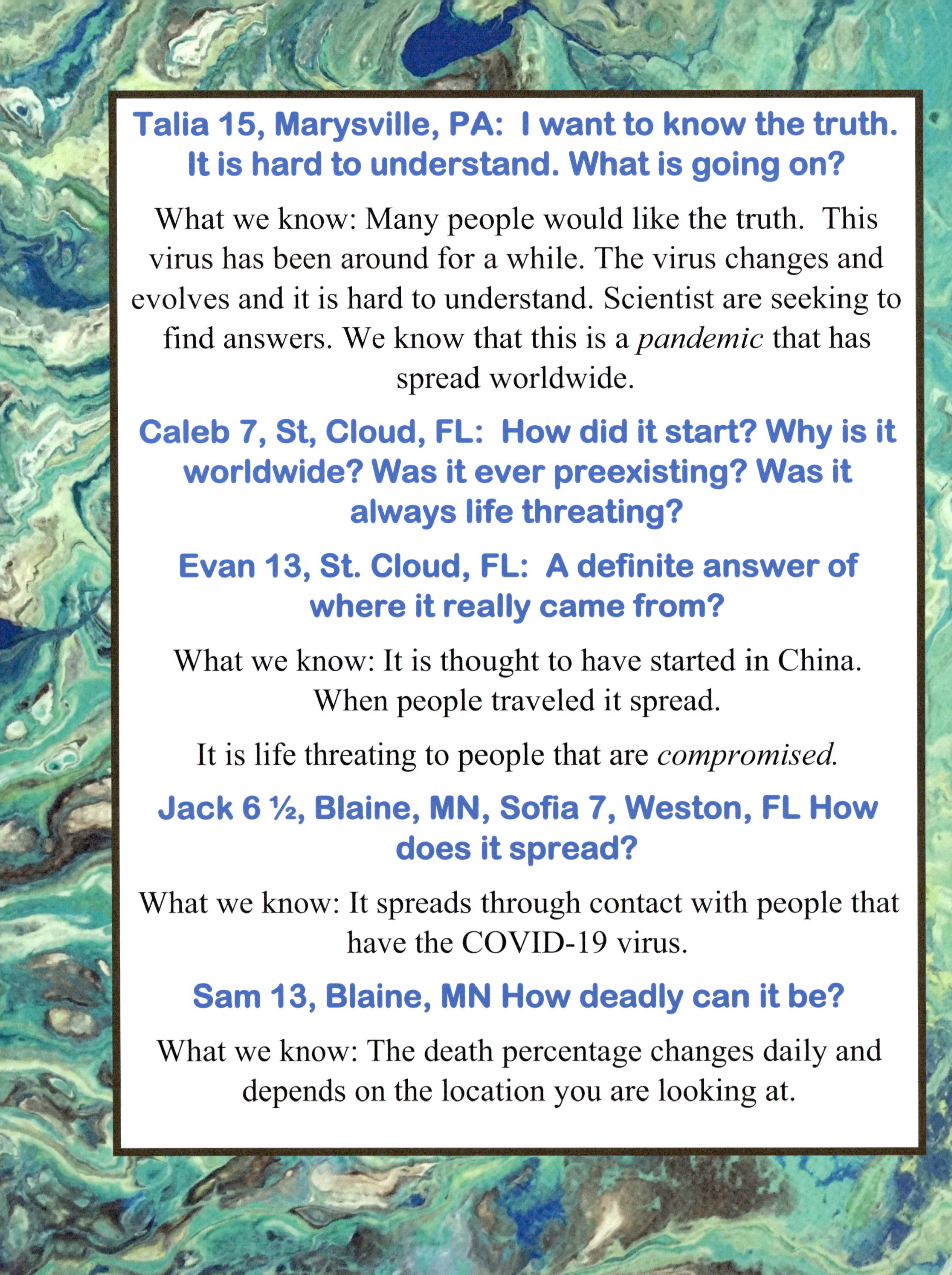


**Talia 15, Marysville, PA:  I want to know the truth. It is hard to understand. What is going on?**

What we know: Many people would like the truth.  This virus has been around for a while. The virus changes and evolves and it is hard to understand. Scientist are seeking to find answers. We know that this is a *pandemic* that has spread worldwide.

**Caleb 7, St, Cloud, FL:  How did it start? Why is it worldwide? Was it ever preexisting? Was it always life threating?**

**Evan 13, St. Cloud, FL:  A definite answer of where it really came from?**

What we know: It is thought to have started in China. When people traveled it spread.

It is life threating to people that are *compromised.*

**Jack 6 ½, Blaine, MN, Sofia 7, Weston, FL How does it spread?**

What we know: It spreads through contact with people that have the COVID-19 virus.

**Sam 13, Blaine, MN How deadly can it be?**

What we know: The death percentage changes daily and depends on the location you are looking at.

What we know: The virus is *mutating* at a slow speed. It is difficult to determine how it is changing. People of all ages can contract the virus.

China has a variety of species of animals and a high concentration of people. These are reason a virus can grow more rapidly.

Diarrhea was not a symptom at first, but later became one. People *hoarded* toilet paper for fear that stores would be closed, and they would not be able to purchase it.



What we know: In adults, the lungs are affected the most with *COVID-19*. In children it is low blood pressure and diarrhea.





What we know: Some people will die from disease. People with underlying conditions and the elderly are the most at risk. Some people may be carriers and show no symptoms.

What we know: It is very *contagious* and spreads through droplets in the air, from a cough or sneeze. *Symptoms* may not appear for 2-3 days after *exposure* to the virus.

The world did not totally shut down. Many countries shut down to contain the virus: but Sweden was one country that remained open.

Children can carry the virus and may have no symptoms, so to keep people with underlying diseases safe, it was recommended that children remain apart to stop the spread of the virus.



What we know: Each school district has their own plan for opening. Many schools are opening in August and September 2020.  Some states are remaining online.

**Kalia 14, St. Cloud, FL:  How to prevent it besides hand sanitizing, washing hands, and what started it?**

What we know: *Vaccines* are being developed as this is written.  Avoid touching your face, nose, and eyes. Wear a mask. Stay six feet apart. Avoid large groups and being in indoors with people you do not live with.

**Emilio 17, St. Cloud, FL:  I want to know how it is spread, like the popcorn theory, like in Italy it does not go from North to South it bounces all over.**

What we know: The spread in Italy, as well as around the world, is partially associated with mobility and linked to different communities and contact with others.

*Contact tracing* refers to finding out who has been affected and whom have them been around. It is gathering information such as have others become infected by the contact or not.

**Trent 6, Shoreview, MN: I hate the virus.**

What we know: You are not alone. Many people are getting tired of being separated from loved ones.

### Mikey 13, St Cloud, FL: How am I going to be affected by it?

What we know: Each person is affected different from the *COVID 19* Virus. Outward aspects, school closings, social distancing, wearing a mask, changes in schedules, and hand washing, sanitizing, small groups, are a few of the changes.

### Mo 14, St. Cloud, FL: How long does it take before you know you have it, so you could stay inside and have groceries delivered?

What we know: Test results for the *COVID-19* virus varies. Some test results can be available in a few hours. Other test results take two to three days; at times, some testing results can take a period of 14 days. It varies depending on the amount of people tested, the place they were tested, and how many results the lab had to process. Recommendations are if you are showing *symptoms*, take the test and quarantine for a period of 14 days, new data now says a period of 10 -14 days of *isolation* after a positive result.

### Alex 15, Saint Cloud, FL Antonius 10, Marana, AZ: Exactly where is started and how? Jarin 18, Saint Cloud, FL:  What is the specific cause of it?

What we know: *World Health Organization* (WHO) identified Wuhan, China as the place of the first outbreak.

The how is still being debated.

**Avery 16, Blaine, MN:  What is the cure or vaccine for the virus? Ceyan 14, St. Cloud, FL: How do we cure it? When should we expect a cure? Is there a cure?**

What we know: *Vaccines* are being released as this is written January 2021. Worldwide it may take to up to 2024 for everyone that wants to be vaccinated to get the *vaccine.*

Forty-nine *vaccines* are being developed around the world (according to www.aprx.org. Dec. 14, 2020).

***Pfizer, Moderna,*** and ***Oxford AstraZeneca***, are a few pharmacies releasing their vaccines in December 2020, and January 2021.

**Gabby Teen: Milaca, MN**

**How do the strains differ, how many are there?**

What we know: Scientists do not agree on number of strains some say one, others report multiple strains. We do know that as of January 2021, there are *mutations or variants* to the *COVID-19* virus, and we are seeing new mutations appear daily.

**Promise 10, Winter Haven, FL: What age can it kill? How many people has it killed?**

What we know: It can kill anyone at any age. People with underlying illness are more likely to have more complications. The number of deaths change daily.

**Abbey 15, St. Cloud, FL:  What is being done to prevent anymore infection a well as what is currently being tested and created for vaccines?**

What we know: *Vaccines* are being developed and some are already being given out to health care workers and the elderly. There are different *vaccines*, with different ingredients.  By April 2021 in the United States,  ages 16 years and older are able to get the vaccine.

Anyone showing any symptoms of *COVID-19* is encouraged to get tested.

**Judah 4, Mount Morris, PA:  I want to know how people get sick from the virus?**

What we know: People get sick if exposed to the virus. *Covid-19* is spread by droplets in the air when people cough, sneeze, talk, or sing.

**Paisley 8, St. Cloud, FL:  What does it look like?   I think it looks like a spikey little ball.**

What we know: The virus under the microscope does look like a spikey ball. It is spherical in shape and covered in bumps or spikes.

What we know: Access to *vaccines* is being sent to high-risk populations, some high-income countries have also agreed to help fund organizations that provide vaccines to the needy countries and people. This is a World-wide pandemic and Countries are learning to work together to help each other.



What we know: Scientist and *pharmaceutical companies* are working hard to create a vaccine that would help stop the spread of the virus. We do not know when it will stop. Vaccines are being given out, but that does not mean it will be stopped. Schools in some places have gone back. Some schools are shutting down again. It depends on governors of each state to determine guidelines, the CDC provides national guidelines for the USA. It spread quickly across the country due to travel and close contact with people infected.

What we know: The teachers stayed at home with their families.  Many started teaching online from home.

The Author loved this response hence the title of this book.

**What do you want to know about the virus?  Write your answer below:**

_______________________________________________
_______________________________________________
_______________________________________________
_______________________________________________
_______________________________________________
_______________________________________________
_______________________________________________
_______________________________________________
_______________________________________________
_______________________________________________
_______________________________________________
_______________________________________________
_______________________________________________
_______________________________________________

# Question 2: What do you want us to know about the virus?

**Elena 6:** You already know everything.

**Sam 6:** It means stay home and be healthy.

**Carmen 9:** It is all around the world.

**Dean 13:** A lot of stores and businesses are closing down. We should take precautions.

**Talia 15:** It is affecting more people that didn't have it.

**Hatcher 13:** Listen to social distancing and do not go to public places or crowded areas unless you have no choice. Even than take precautions. Don't risk your loved ones, visits can wait. Use *Skype* or other video chats for visiting. That being said, we have gone on hikes, and have explored nature. We rode our bikes and gone skateboarding. Fresh air is good, just think of ways to enjoy it that keep you at a safe distance from others.

**Hayden 15:** I don't want people to over-react to the situation, as it only seems to escalate the issues. If everyone stays calm and keeps level-headed the storm will pass. It's not political, it's not racist, and it's not empathetic. It's an ugly virus that can and will affect us all. So, let's help each other get through this. Be neighborly and understand it is not just affecting health, but jobs, schools, and even housing too.

**Jake 12:** Bored from being quarantined.

**Abbey 15:** I would like others to know that though it is a virus like the flu it is worse and a worldwide pandemic.

**Avery 16:** Fine as the virus has not reached me.

**Blake 14:** Fine, bored.

**Jonah 17:** I am doing good, it is boring, but we are doing good.

**Jack 5 ½ and Sam 13:** Nothing

**Promise 10:** It can possibly even be in the neighborhood or in Winter Haven.

**Emilio 17:** I would like people to know how severe it is and the precautions. If they don't take precautions it really affects others.

**Alex 15:** Better ways to prepare for it and prevent it from getting too their kids.

**Mikey 13:** How to keep everyone safe from it.

**Mo 14:** I know it originated in China and spread throughout the world by traveling.

**Evan 13:** I want to let people to know about, Social interactions, not to pass it. Separate from one another.

**Kalia 14:** How to better protect the children.

**Mila 2:** Daddy is helping people at work.

**Trent 6:** It is stupid.

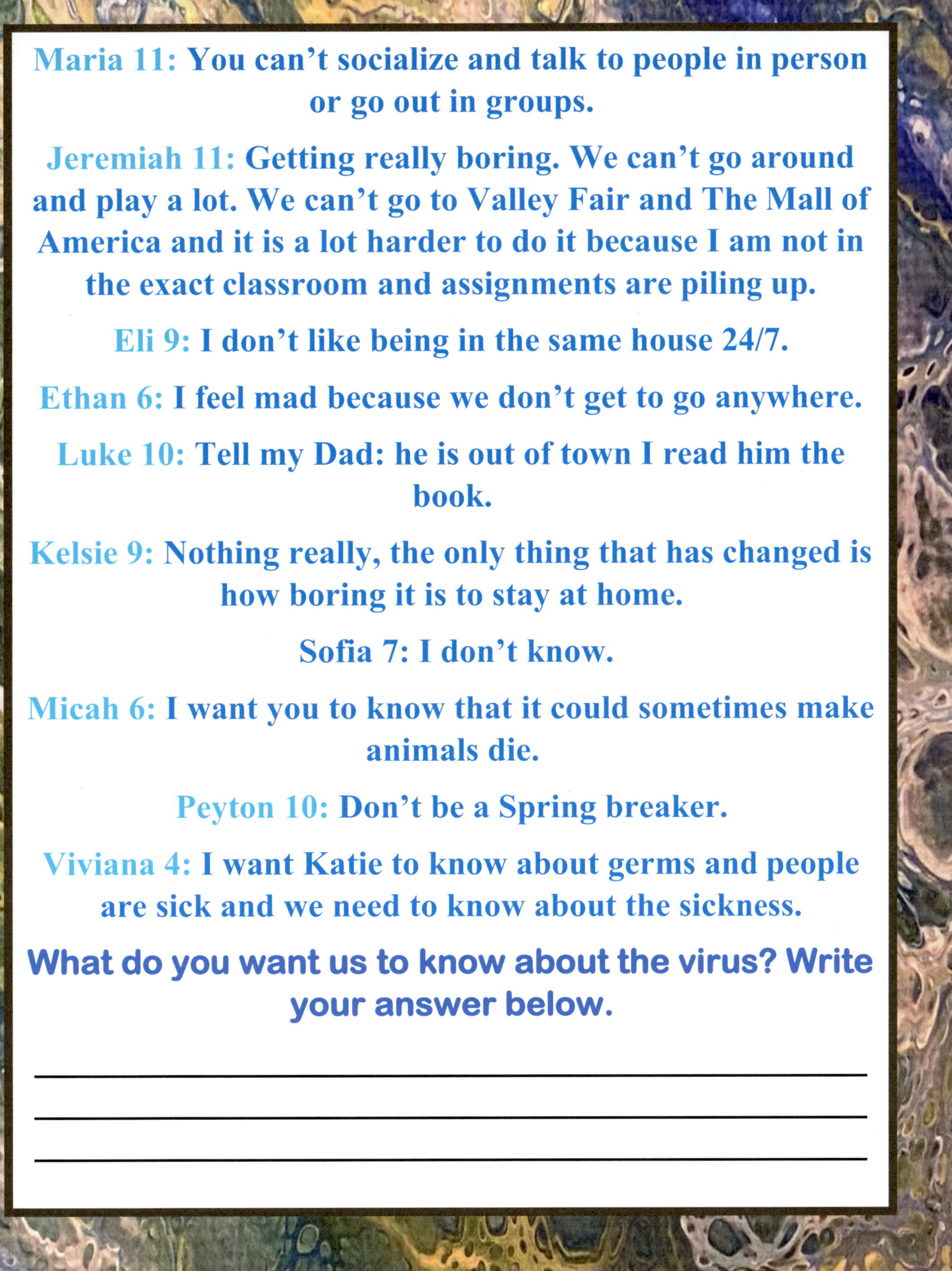

**Maria 11:** You can't socialize and talk to people in person or go out in groups.

**Jeremiah 11:** Getting really boring. We can't go around and play a lot. We can't go to Valley Fair and The Mall of America and it is a lot harder to do it because I am not in the exact classroom and assignments are piling up.

**Eli 9:** I don't like being in the same house 24/7.

**Ethan 6:** I feel mad because we don't get to go anywhere.

**Luke 10:** Tell my Dad: he is out of town I read him the book.

**Kelsie 9:** Nothing really, the only thing that has changed is how boring it is to stay at home.

**Sofia 7:** I don't know.

**Micah 6:** I want you to know that it could sometimes make animals die.

**Peyton 10:** Don't be a Spring breaker.

**Viviana 4:** I want Katie to know about germs and people are sick and we need to know about the sickness.

**What do you want us to know about the virus? Write your answer below.**

_______________________________________________

_______________________________________________

_______________________________________________

# Question 3: <u>How are you doing?</u>

**Dean 13:** I am fine I have not caught anything yet.

**Elena 6:** Fine because I am not old.

**Carmen 9:** Good, but I was sick yesterday, I was a bit dizzy. I feel good now.

**Viviana 4, Ethan 6, Trent 6, Micah 6, Sofia 7, Joey 7, Sydney 6, Sam 13:** Good!

**Jarin 18:** Alright. Staying at home, doing online homework so I can get into college.

**Elias 5:** Terrific!

**Judah 4:** A little bit good.

**Caleb 7:** Scared, I am scared that there's so much close to us, so I don't want it to get us. That is why I am scared. I feel like it is scary outside when I'm near people, so I go far around them if I am on my bike.

**Paisley 8:** Umm…good. I am sad, umm bored, and scared. I am good because I get to be home with my family. I feel sad because there's a lot of families losing people and they can't go to the church for the funeral. I'm not really mad or miserable. I'm bored because I usually tell jokes and play really fun games with my friends, but sometimes those games don't make sense to my brothers and they don't get the jokes I play with my friends.

**Ceyan 14:** Let's see…I feel really bad for the people that have it and are dying. I feel bad for the workers. I hope they're well and their families are okay. I just need to think that we're all in this together. I'm kind of bored because I have nothing much going on right now, but I don't have it as bad as people who are working or sick right now. I should be grateful that I'm healthy and my family is healthy as well, but I am also pretty bored right now.

**Nate 12:** It's pretty scary. Not really because of the pandemic, but because there's a lot of people without income right now and even when it ends it'll be pretty scary. The lasting effects of the pandemic scare me.

**Victor 14, Alex 15:** Good.

**Antonius 10:** I am doing good, no experience with it. I am sure some are bound to have it soon.

**Abbey 15:** I am doing well. I have been enjoying extra free time, and not having to wake up early.

**Jake 12:** I am doing well because it is nice to rest.

**Jack 5 ½:** Good. I don't even have the Corona virus.

**Blake 14:** Fine. Bored.

**Jonah 17:** I am doing good. It is boring but we are doing good.

**Avery 16:** Fine as the virus has not reached me.

**Emilio 17:** I am physically o.k. Mentally frustrated about what it is doing to people.  Mortality rate not that high. I am a senior and prom and celebrations, I worked for 12 years for, won't happen. I am an AP student, and we worked our butts off to get good grades and now they are canceling it, we now have to take it at home and our chances are less.

**Mikey 13:** I am o.k.

**Mo 14:** I am doing good. Not much changed, although I am scared because some people are insane.

**Evan 13:** Mad, it happened during Spring break and I can't do anything, but I am trying to deal with it.

**Kalia 14:** Well o.k. It just feels weird not being able to leave the house.

**Mila 2:** Sad you can't go to the park. It is dirty.

**Jeremiah 11:** Kind of good.

**Talia 15:** I am o.k. I am good because I have done well. I am healthy, exercising, and staying away from others, I am a little shaken up from it.

**Peyton 10:** Good, Thank you!

**Kelsie 10:** Good I just miss my friends. It is sad.

**Sam 6:** Great!

**Maria 11:** I am doing good; I am just really bored because it is not easy to talk to your friends or see them. **Teachers:** Be safe and make sure you have enough supplies. **Classmates:** I miss some of them and I hope we can see each other in May (2020).

**Hatcher 13:** I am doing fine, but our community is affected, stores going out of stock, restaurants closing, or switching to delivery or curbside pickup only and our streets are quiet there is less traffic.  A big positive I have noticed neighbors helping each other, There have been people sitting in their driveways and waving at others who are taking walks or riding bikes. No one is getting close but just being good neighbors and watching out for each other, I can see a positive change in the way it is bring the community closer.

**Hayden 15:** I am doing o.k. I wish I could see my friends, but I thank god we live in a digital age. I can at least chat, play video games, and have video facetime with friends and family near and far.

**How are you doing? Write your answer below:**

_______________________________________________

_______________________________________________

_______________________________________________

_______________________________________________

# Question 4:  <u>What do you want to tell your friends, classmates, and teachers?</u>

Sam 6: I miss my friends and teachers.

Elena 6: The virus is not dangerous because we are not old.

Carmen 9: I call them on the phone and get facetime. Classmates: still study.

Sofia 7: I don't know.

Micah 6: The virus can make you really sick.

Jarin 18: Stay home and stay safe. Teachers: This year has been fun, and I hope to see them in the near future. Classmates: Stay home.

Elias 5: Do any of you have the Corona virus? I am sorry if you have the virus but please think of me because I miss you.

Judah 4: I love you and hope you have a good day. I am very sorry the Corona virus is here and I'm sorry you can't go outside. I pray for you to get better in no time if you get sick.

Ceyan 14: We will make it through this. Just have faith. I miss you. I miss hanging out with you and playing video games in school. I miss having my teachers there to instruct me rather than online. I miss face-to-face contact. I miss school in general, seeing all the people that are not my family.

Nate 12: (Singing) We're all in this together. We may be socially distanced, but our hearts beat as one.

Paisley 8: I miss them, Yeah, I miss them.

Antonius 10: Young and old stay in.  The kids are not going to get sick, but you could spread it to your parents. Teachers and classmates:  Stay home and stay active.

Abbey 15: I would like to tell others to be safe and try to limit contact with others.

Jake 12: Wish they were safe.

Avery 16: I would ask them things, if they kept weightlifting or are doing body workouts at home?

Jonah 17: Stay inside it is not easy, you get everyone else sick and could die. Teachers: It has been a nice three weeks without you. Classmates: Stay inside and wash your hands.

Sam 13: Try not to be around people stay in your house and be healthy.

Jack 5 ½: It has spread around the world. Teachers: I don't really like staying home a lot.

Blake 14:

Promise 10: Don't be scared if we have it, we won't die, and Jesus is always protecting us. Teachers: When we go back to school if one has it, stay 6 feet away, it will be o.k. Classmates: One if us in the household can have it, we shouldn't be scared about it, if one of us has it the hospital will take care of us.

**Emilio 17:** *Quarantine* and maintain good hygiene, keep that Social distancing, and don't give in to peer pressure. Teachers, I am proud of you and your hard work. Without your ambition of making students feel better, the hope would be gone.  Classmates: It is not the end.  Keep the hope, you will have Prom and Graduation and if we don't have Prom. We will have graduation the most important.

**Alex 15:** If everyone in your family is o.k. and no one has gotten sick? Teachers, thank you for sending messages and being lenient, so we could get our work done.

**Mikey 13:** Be careful and stay inside. Teachers: be safe. Classmates: be careful and don't spread anything.

**Mo 14:** Stay inside and not have people over.

**Evan 13:** I am doing good, and I am not sick.

**Kalia 14:** I want to see you again and not have to worry about this COVID-19 when things are back too normal. I miss them. Teachers: hope you are doing well, and I will get to see them again someday, I miss them.  Classmates, I hope you have not gotten COVID-19 and I hope you are taking care of them.

**Ethan 6:** How the Corona virus stop? Teachers: how did the Corona virus get created?

**Hayden 15:** I miss you, but we will be back too normal soon. So, stay safe and be careful. Listen to advisors so we can beat this faster and get back to normal.

**Trent 6:** I hate the virus and I want to kill the virus. Teachers: I like school. Classmates: I want to tell the kids I hate COVID.

**Mila 2:** They are at the houses. Be careful.

**Viviana 4:** I can't tell my friends, because my grandpa and family doesn't know my friends. I am fine. Classmates: I can't tell them because of the sickness. They have the sickness.

**Jeremiah 11:** Kind of good. It is getting boring, and I don't like sitting at home. I miss playing with them and hanging around with them. Teachers: I miss being in the classroom.

**Eli 9:** Did you have a cold in the past two weeks? I miss playing football. Should we have new teams? Teachers: I miss being in my class. I am glad I get taught. I like to learn from all my teachers.  Classmates: I am glad I can be back in class and not work alone.

**Luke 10:** I can't go to school until 5$^{th}$ grade.

**Payton 10:** Stay home.

**Kelsie 9:** We can talk to them and we talk about how weird it is we can't play with our friends, it is sad. Classmates: I miss them.

**Dean 13:** Stay at home, stay safe, don't go out too much, and no large gatherings. Classmates: They are not online so I can't tell them much.

**Victor 14:** That I miss them, and I hope they are staying safe.

**Talia 15:** I miss them, and I hope they are doing well and taking the right precautions.

**Hatcher 13:** I want them to stay safe, take cautions in public areas and stay in contact with your family, make sure they are safe, and have what they need. If you are bored, use this time to learn something that school does not teach you, like how to make a cake from scratch, change a flat tire on a bike or car, help your mom with spring cleaning, or even learn to play in instrument. We live in a digital age and can find all sorts of lessons online.

**Jake 12:** Wish they were safe. son to another person.

**Maria 11:** How quickly it can spread from one per

**Caleb 7:** That I miss them so much and I hope they're doing good and that I hope they're being careful.

## What would you like to tell your friends, teachers, and classmates?  Write it below:

_______________________________________________
_______________________________________________
_______________________________________________
_______________________________________________
_______________________________________________
_______________________________________________
_______________________________________________
_______________________________________________

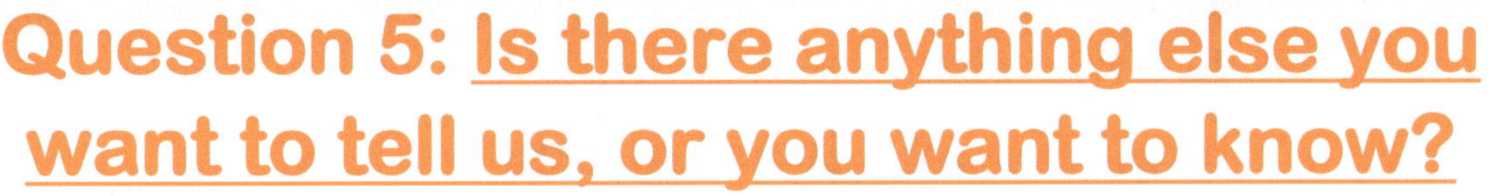

# Question 5: <u>Is there anything else you want to tell us, or you want to know?</u>

**Sam 6:** WASH YOUR HANDS!

**Sofia 7:** How contagious it is.

**Elias 5:** I want to have a big party for my birthday and invite all my cousins and friends, like 25 people.

**Judah 4:** I hope my dad never gets sick because I love him.

**Abbey 15:** I would like to tell others to stay home. Do not buy extra products when you don't need them.

As for classmates, good luck with virtual schooling.

**Victor 14:** How it is affecting jobs and how many people it's helping, and not helping, it's ruining their lives.

**Talia 15, Jonah 17, Antonius 10:** No that is about it.

**Blake 14:** Does age matter on how bad you get it?

**Jack 5 ½:** What does the Corona virus actually do?

**Sam 13:** What is the death percentage?

**Nate 12:** I hope everything can go back to normal.

**Joey 7, Sydney 6:** We want it to be over so we can see all the characters at the theme parks.

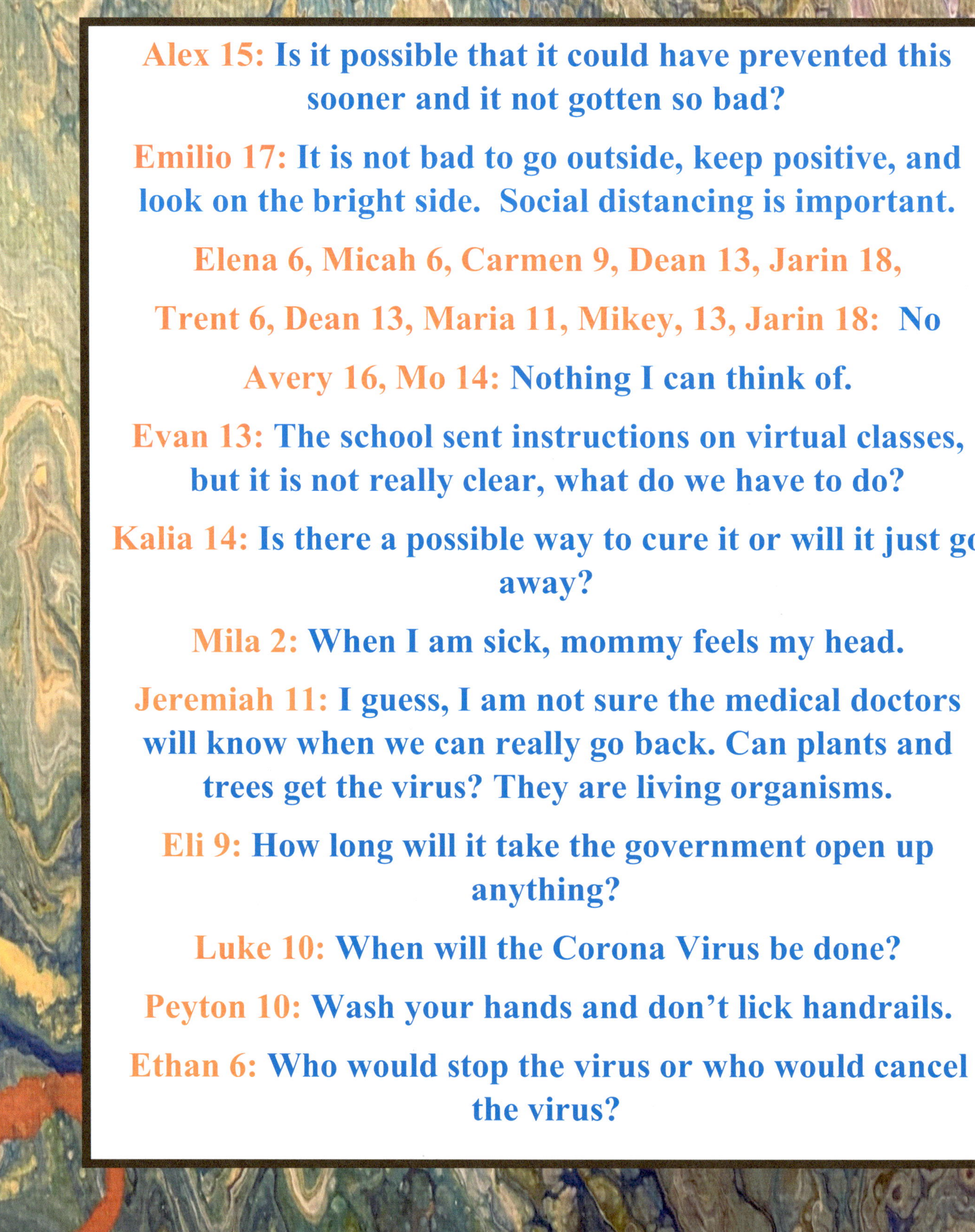

**Alex 15:** Is it possible that it could have prevented this sooner and it not gotten so bad?

**Emilio 17:** It is not bad to go outside, keep positive, and look on the bright side.  Social distancing is important.

**Elena 6, Micah 6, Carmen 9, Dean 13, Jarin 18, Trent 6, Dean 13, Maria 11, Mikey, 13, Jarin 18:**  No

**Avery 16, Mo 14:** Nothing I can think of.

**Evan 13:** The school sent instructions on virtual classes, but it is not really clear, what do we have to do?

**Kalia 14:** Is there a possible way to cure it or will it just go away?

**Mila 2:** When I am sick, mommy feels my head.

**Jeremiah 11:** I guess, I am not sure the medical doctors will know when we can really go back. Can plants and trees get the virus? They are living organisms.

**Eli 9:** How long will it take the government open up anything?

**Luke 10:** When will the Corona Virus be done?

**Peyton 10:** Wash your hands and don't lick handrails.

**Ethan 6:** Who would stop the virus or who would cancel the virus?

**Promise 10:** Don't be scared if we have it, we won't die, and Jesus is always protecting us.

**Hatcher 13:** If you think you may have the virus, self-isolate, call your doctor, wear a mask. Avoid sharing touched items and monitor your symptoms. Drink lots of water and know it won't last forever. We have amazing Doctors, Scientists out there working on vaccine and cure, to help us.

**Kelsie 9:** I really do miss my dad because I don't get to see him when he works. I only see him on weekends.

**Hayden 15:** I am proud of my teacher for doing this, and I am glad to be a part of it, I hope it helps calm anyone who is scared, or unsure of the changes we are living through. The whole world is going through this and I pray it brings us closer together and unifies us all, a little more!   P.S. The roads are less crowded which is making my drivers permit training much more pleasant.

**Caleb 7:** I hope in the future it will end and everything will get back to normal and I won't have to worry about anything anymore and right now all we can do is pray.

**Paisley 8:** When it ends it's going to be like it's a whole new world. Like we feel like we're the first people outside because the world is going to feel so different once it ends.

**Ceyan 14:** We just got to be strong in our hearts. We WILL make it through this together.

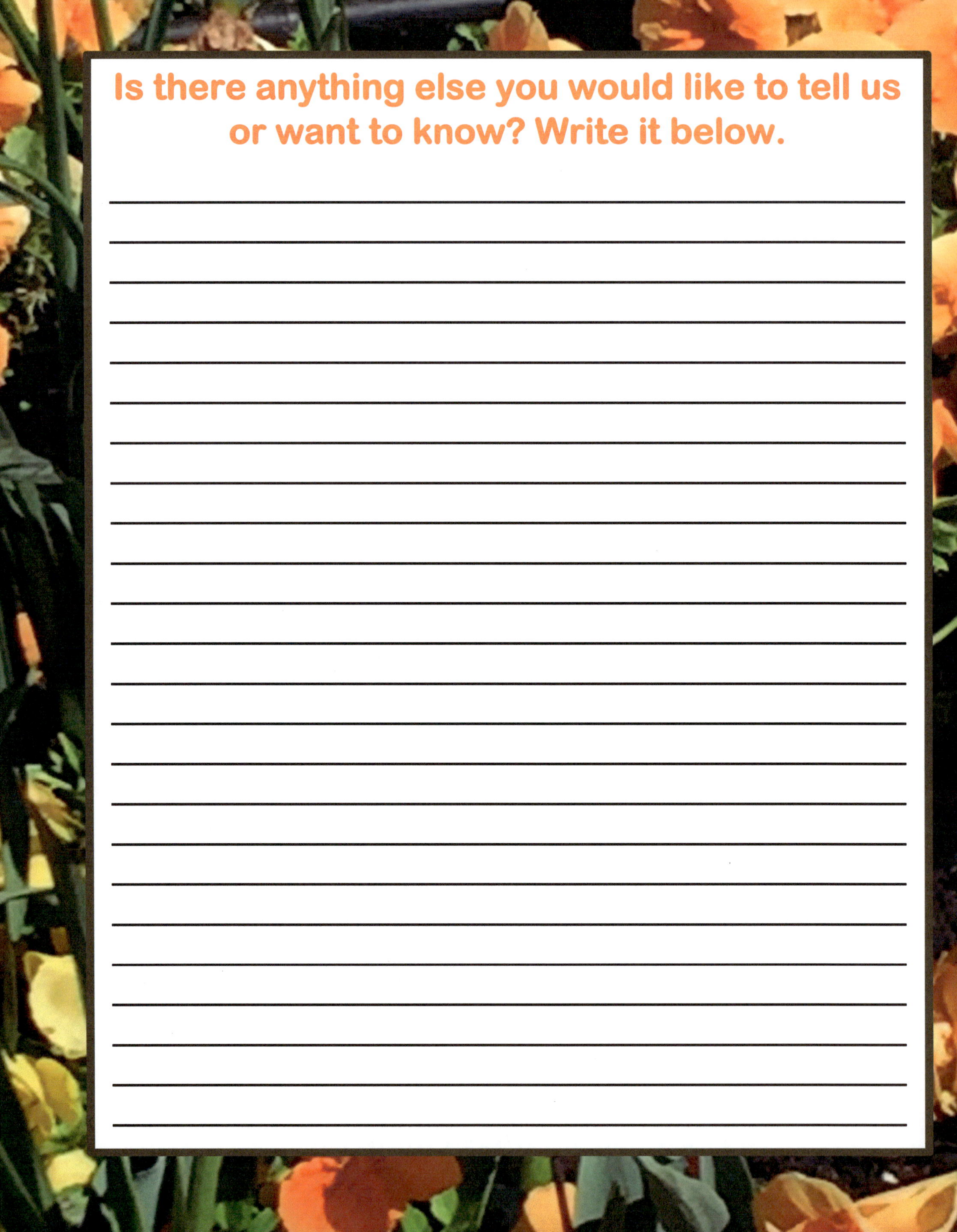


Is there anything else you would like to tell us or want to know? Write it below.

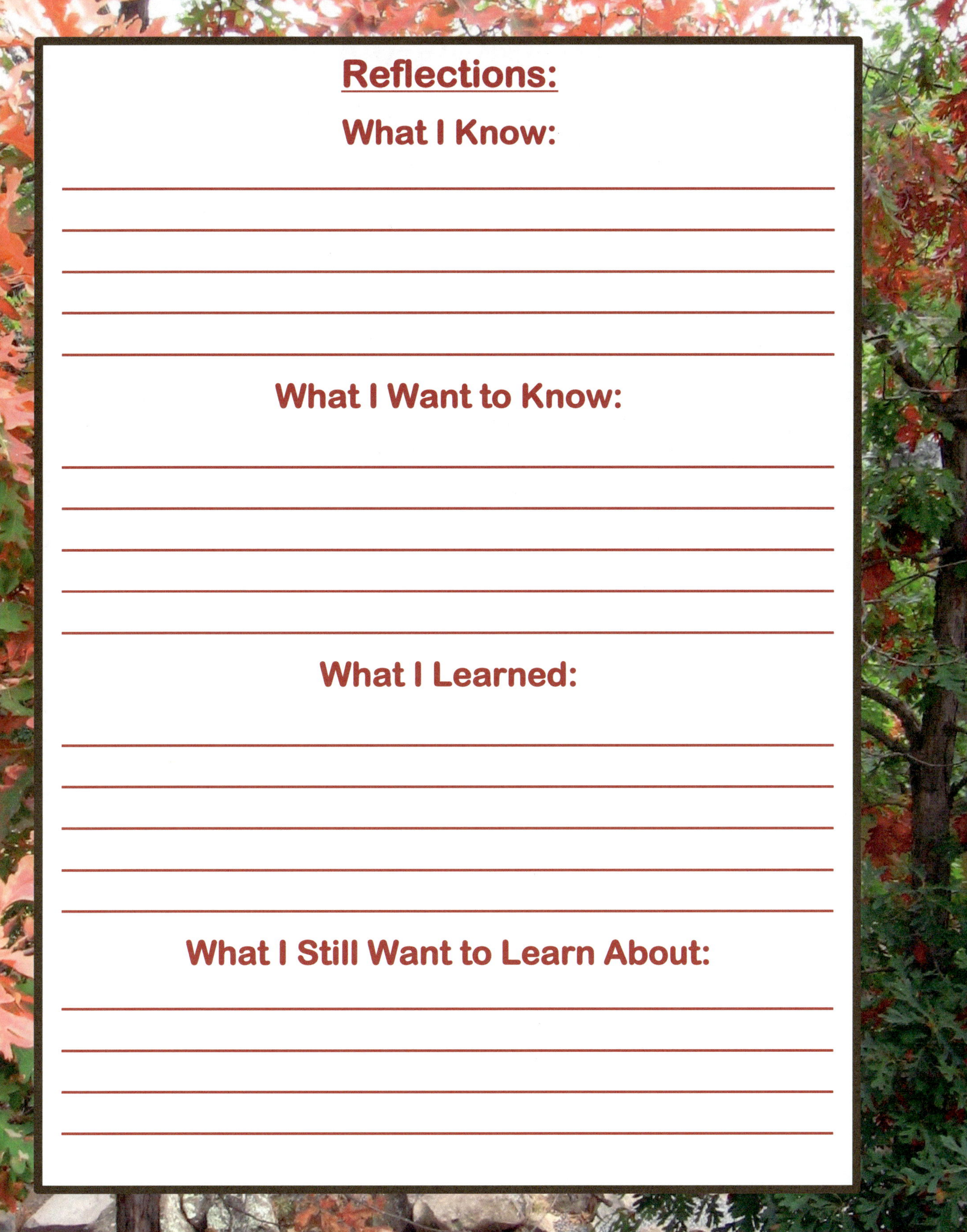

Reflections:
What I Know:
What I Want to Know:
What I Learned:
What I Still Want to Learn About:

# Vocabulary A-H

***Asymptomatic:*** Shows no symptoms for the illness you may have.

***Compromised Health:*** Has an under-lying condition that causes a person to have a higher chance of getting an illness.

***Contact Tracing:*** Follows people that have an illness, in this case, COVID-19 and lets people know if they have been exposed to the virus.

***Contagious:*** Someone that has an illness that can expose and transmit the disease to others.

***Coronavirus:*** A disease that may have symptoms that appear 2-14 days after exposure.

***COVID-19****: Another name for Coronavirus.*

***Exposure:*** *Coming into contact with someone that has tested positive for the disease or illness.*

***Evolves:*** Changes over time.

***Fatigue:*** Tired or exhausted.

***Hoarding:*** Collecting or saving items more than is needed.

## Words You Want to Know:

______________________________________________

______________________________________________

______________________________________________

# Vocabulary I-Z

***Immune System:*** The part of your body that fights infections.

***Isolation:*** Separating people who are sick from healthy people.

***Mutate:*** Changes over time.

***Obesity:*** Having excessive body fat.

***Oxygen Levels:*** The amount of oxygen in your blood.

***Pandemic:*** Disease or illness that spreads quickly across many countries.

***Pharmaceutical Companies:*** Companies that make medications.

***Quarantine:*** Limiting movement and exposure to others.

***Respiratory:*** Breathing

***Symptoms:*** Signs that you have a possible illness.

***Vaccination:*** A shot, spray, or mixture given to prevent or lessen a disease.

***Virus:*** An infection that can be transmitted to people or plants, and/or animals.

## Words You Want to Know:

_______________________________________

_______________________________________

_______________________________________

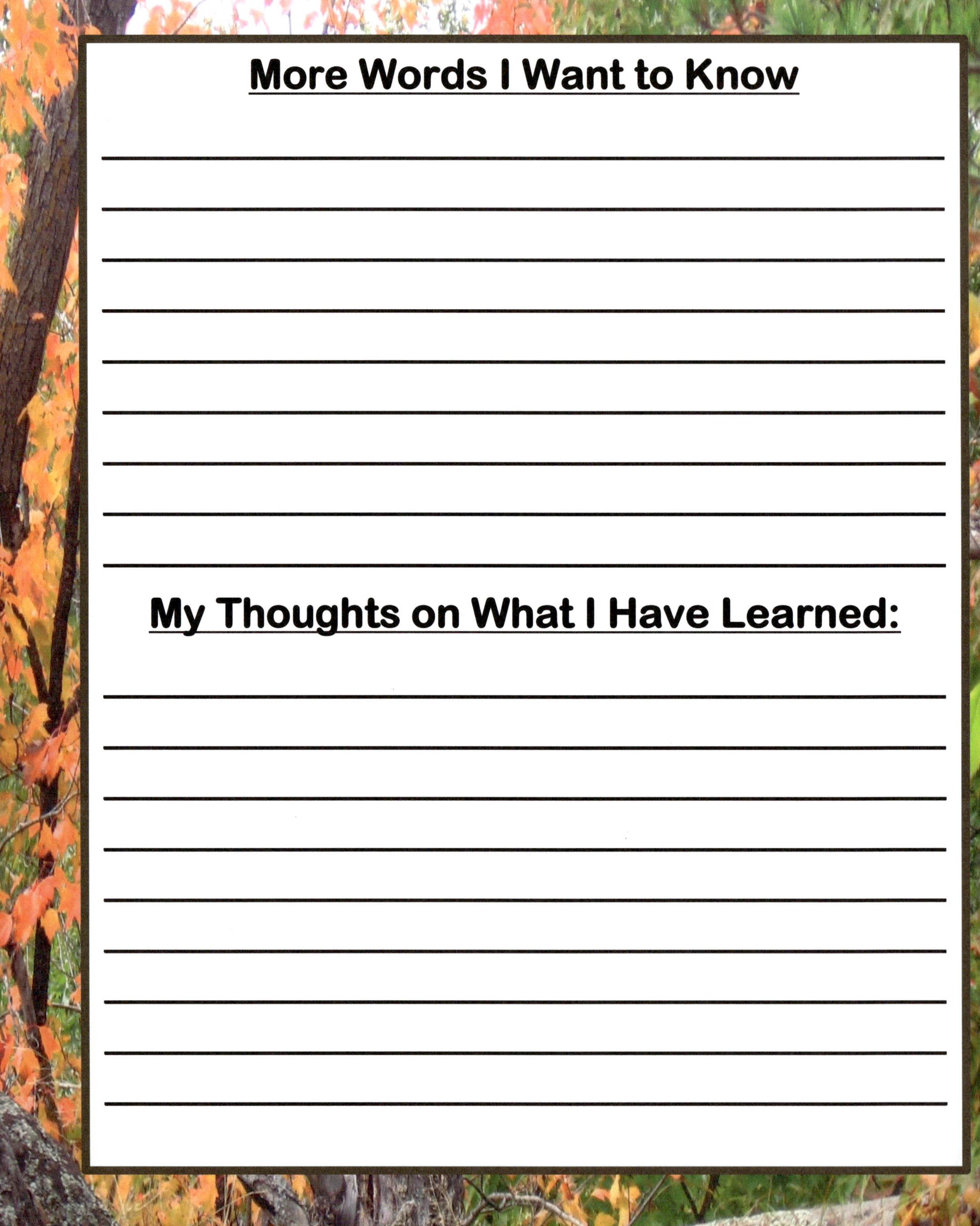

More Words I Want to Know

My Thoughts on What I Have Learned:

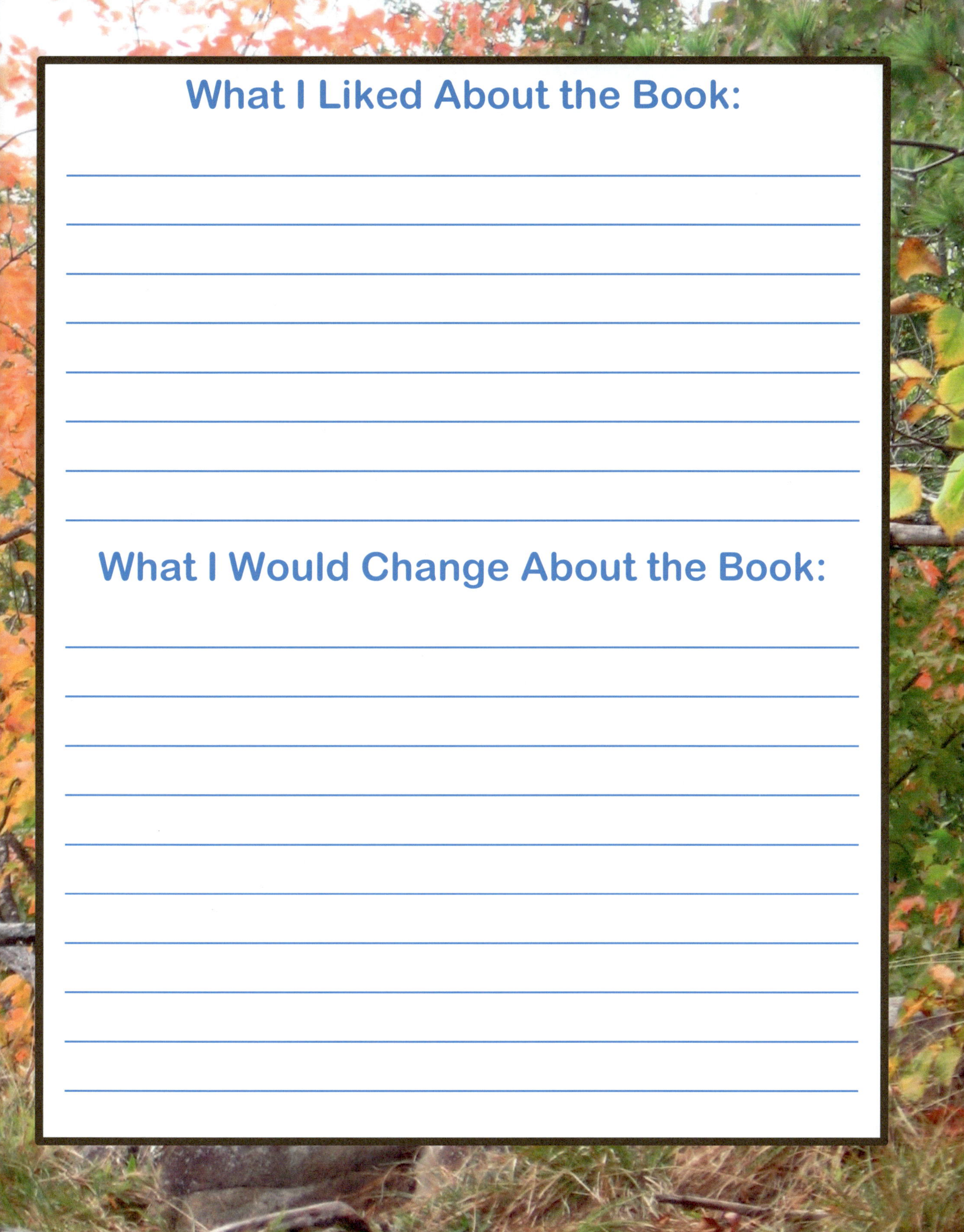

What I Liked About the Book:

What I Would Change About the Book:

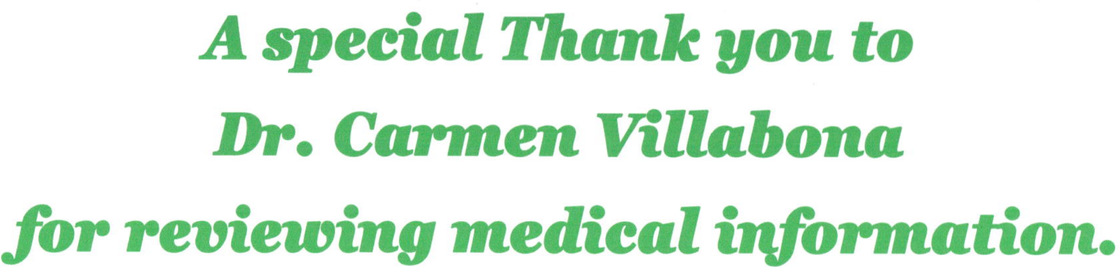



## Websites used in research:

https://www.cdc.gov/coronavirusdisease2019

*https://www.childrensmn.org/2020/05/19/multisystem-inflammatory-syndrome-children-associated-covid-19/

https://www.npr.org/sections/health-shots/2020/10/05/920446534/cdc-acknowledges-coronavirus-can-spread-via-airborne-transmission

https://www.who.int/coronavirusdisease

Questions and responses based on research and CDC reports, Medical Reviews, and are not necessarily the views of the Author. Children's answers are in their own words. Slight changes may have been made for the sake of understanding. Ages of children were at the time of interviews:

Winter 2020

Made in the USA
Monee, IL
07 July 2026